Acts of Attention: The Poems of D.H. Lawrence

In The Fourth World: Poems

Emily's Bread: Poems

The Madwoman in the Attic:
The Woman Writer and the 19th Century Literary Imagination
(with Susan Gubar)

No Man's Land:
The Place of the Woman Writer in the 20th Century
(with Susan Gubar)

Shakespeare's Sisters:
Feminist Essays on Women Poets
(editor, with Susan Gubar)

The Norton Anthology of Literature by Women:
The Tradition in English
(editor, with Susan Gubar)

Blood Pressure

W · W · NORTON & COMPANY · NEW YORK · LONDON

Blood Pressure

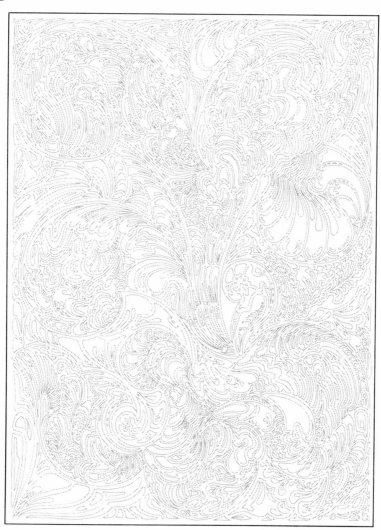

Sandra M. Gilbert

Published simultaneously in Canada by Penguin Books Canada Ltd.,
2801 John Street, Markham, Ontario L3R 1B4.
Printed in the United States of America.

The text of this book is composed in Avanta, with display type set in L S C Condensed.
Composition and Manufacturing by The Haddon Craftsmen, Inc. Book design by
Antonina Krass.

First Edition

Library of Congress Cataloging-in-Publication Data

Gilbert, Sandra M.
    Blood pressure
        p. cm.
    I. Title.
    PS3557.I34227B55   1988
    811'.54—dc 19   88-5873

ISBN 0-393-02609-4

W. W. Norton & Company, Inc., 500 Fifth Avenue, New York, N. Y. 10110
W. W. Norton & Company Ltd., 37 Great Russell Street, London WC1B 3NU

1 2 3 4 5 6 7 8 9 0

Acknowledgments

Some of these poems (a few in slightly different form) have appeared in the following journals:

The American Scholar: "Late Beethoven"

Beloit Poetry Journal: "A Year Later"

Field: "The Last Poem About the Snow Queen," "Accident," "Pinocchio," "The Parachutist's Wife"

Iowa Review: "You Fall," "You Meet the Real Dream Mother-in-Law," "You Discover You're in Love with the Dead Prince," "The One He Loves," "The Love Sickness," "The Cure"

Massachusetts Review: "The Return of the Muse," "The Summer Kitchen"

Missouri Review: "Grandpa," "2085," "Hooked Rug"

Poetry: "Thinking About an Old Friend," "Blood Pressure," "To a Man Who Advises Maturity," "Rissem," "My Grandmother in Paris," "The Mothers at Seventy," "In the Golden *Sala,*" "For Miss Lewis and Miss Newton," "After Thanksgiving," "Rain/Insomnia/North Coast"

Poetry Northwest: "Phaeton," "This Is Not . . . ," "New Year's Eve," "Low Tide," "Beets"

Poetry Now: "Five Potatoes"

Ontario Review: "Singles, or, Never Eat Standing Up," "Reproduction," "Empty Nest," "Marriage"

Prairie Schooner: "The Three Sisters"

Thirteenth Moon: "What He Hates/What He Loves"

Three Penny Review: "Jackson Heights"

Woman/Poet: "The Twelve Dancing Princesses"

In addition, "The Summer Kitchen," "Beets," and "Five Potatoes" appeared in 1984 as part of a chapbook entitled *The Summer Kitchen,* published by the Heyeck Press, Woodside, California.

Finally, I am grateful to Frank Bidart, Robert Fagles, Susan Gubar, Diana O Hehir, Robert Pinsky, Ruth Stone, and Alan Williamson for their encouragement, friendship, and advice.

again, for Elliot

Contents

III The Summer Kitchen

IV The Parachutist's Wife

I
The Love Sequence

You Discover You're in Love
With the Dead Prince

You thought, He must be pale, he must be silent,
he must sit by the river all morning gazing at nothing.
And when he sat on the bank, his eyes focused on nothing,
you thought, It's me he sees in the middle distance,
he's watching my dance, he's in love
with the dance of my invisible bones.

For him you turned your skin to cream.
You thought, he'll sip my body like a spirit
potion, and come to the secret
place of my heart—for he's the one
who loves my eyelids, he's the one
who bathes his wrist in the cold stream
because he dreams of the blue vein behind my ankle.

And all the time he was dead, he was the boy king
in the coffin of ice, the one with the mirror splinter
caught in his left eye, the royal child
attended by women and mourners,
whose long trance was demanded, they said, by mystic
signs from the stars.

                    In his dead cellar,
among the jewels and mirrors,
the sacred nurses feed him cream through tubes,
they bathe his silence in sweet wine.
All night a fire of thorny twigs
flickers cold, cold. . . .

You looked into the pale flames. You watched
the ceremonies of shadow. You wept.
You said you couldn't believe it.
You said, O prince, O friend, O lover,
climb out of that snowdrift
and come to this meadow where the blackberries ripen
and the bees hum like summer.

And he smiled in his trance, and said,
What snowdrift? What meadow? What summer?

How You Fell

You were the proud one, the kid in the secret room
lit by organdy curtains white as milk,
the one who had a special destiny
inscribed on her forehead with invisible ink.

April evenings sparrows lined up on your fire escape
to tell you their tales of old verandahs,
palm trees, Florida afternoons:
you were going to walk on warm sands, marry

the master of the plantation, command
the fountain that gushed wine.
Love would rain on you like geranium balm, love
would fortify your heart against everyone

except the one who was just, the one who loved you
more than his own bones, the one
whose beard shone in the wind
like the wild grass behind the schoolyard.

Who took you to the door of the oven?
Who walked you into the cooking pot? Who
introduced you to the vizier of silence with his
wand of ice, his cape of dead leaves?

You knew he'd enlisted under a blank banner, knew
he was missing crucial fingers, knew
he was the agent for somebody else.
But it didn't matter, you stayed put,

you baked in the cave of change,
your hair dampened, your
secret organs hummed with love.
When you came out,

he turned toward you, his pale gaze fell on you
like the headlights of a dark car
rounding a bend on an empty road at midnight.

He told you how little you mattered.

Behind him you heard the sea
falling and falling on terrible rocks.

You were sticky and thick with love
like the broken windowpane the witch painted over with sugar.

You Meet the Real
Dream Mother-in-Law

In the anteroom of silence you waited to meet
the dream mother-in-law,
fingering old magazines, their exhausted edges, the places
where recipes were torn away. . . .

You sat straight as a washboard in your
naugahyde chair, holding your breath,
never complaining: you knew
she was in there and how it would be—

the long still room with bloodcolored rugs,
the tables on eighteenth-century stilts, the hair
Atlantic gray, the bone china cups
with blue frost, the silvertipped cane, the misty

voice of Ethel Barrymore, saying,
I've waited so long, *he's* waited so long,
but how glad we are, my dear,
that you're the one!

And then the talk would unfold like fine lace,
the talk of women who'd take a lifetime
to trace this intricate design. . . .
Silk the color of tea leaves, fingers keen as crystal,

she'd love your sonnets, give you
sherry that had slept in the cabinet
since her impudent sister ran off with that
mean metaphysician: she'd

want you to have her grandmother's sapphire,
tell you legends of sombre attics,
clasp your hand between ivory gloves
and make you hers, hers. . . .

When they opened the double doors and led you in,
you were surprised to find a naked waitress
sulking on a shell-shaped sofa.

Her son winked and blew poison darts at you
like the bad kid next door, the one
who was always stoned on something rotten.

She accused you of doing wicked things in the dark,
told you to hurry up and start sorting grain, said
you should remember there was a mountain you'd have to climb.

You stared like a fool at her granite breasts, her great
snowy belly, her whole
ferocious body.

   Smoke
curled from between her thighs
like the awful breath of factories.

You Call Him Little Kay,
You Sing Him an Aubade

Kay sat quite alone in all those many miles of empty ice halls.
. . . He sat so stiff and immovable that one might have
thought he was frozen to death.

— Hans Christian Andersen, "The Snow Queen"

Dawn is when you think of him
in his frostblue cave,
your little Kay, with the sand of
disbelief in his eye:

His coma isn't over,
in his trance he dreams
equations of ice, crosswords, night wine
he sucks from the Snow Queen's nipples.

But clarity comes in from the sea:
the fierce morning, a freckled girl
in a glass dress, tells
about breakers, tells

about light far out,
blue-green light that
makes a raft of brilliance
lovers float on. . . .

You want to smash the heavy doors of his chamber!
Slide the velvet curtains open with a clang!

That eager girl will come in flashing.
The gold of her rings

will dance across his eyelids:
in his sleep

he'll hear her whisper, he'll
smile, he'll spit out all that darkness
and grow strong new arms
to hug her with.

The One He Loves

She's the figure skater you've always hated,
the princess of the spelling bee, the ice queen
in velvet and fur
with muscles tough as tusks
and hair the color of charm bracelets.

Next to her you're flabby and noisy, something
made of jelly instead of sinew,
something that shivers and whimpers
and passes out in the dark, a princess of pain
with weak ankles and a head full of misspelled sentences.

Once you asked her the secret: how do you
always keep your skates on, how do you memorize
the whole dictionary? She smiled and talked too slowly,
a native telling a foreigner
the way through some inexplicable city.

In the palace of his mind
they reign forever on twin frost thrones.
Suave servants in black and white
circle them like gulls, offering trays
on which odd canapés swarm thick as wishes.

She nibbles, royal, muscular, silent.
He watches, a furtive cat on the edge of shadow:
he wants her to burn his skin, wants her
to crack his bones, wants the fine spray from her skates
to baptize his wrists like radioactive sleet.

11

Around them expensive dancers loop and spin.
She and he yawn, hum, play chess, play Scrabble.
A cold flame flickers between them
on polished granite; only they
know what it means, only they.

The Love Sickness

You lie on the sofa all day, washed in fog,
your heart twittering like a thrush among prickly branches.
You think you're that last black tree before the beach, the one
that trembles so close to the cliff edge it seems to have
one toe in the abyss. . . .

Your toes are dissolving like that, your whole body
melting and thinning, becoming transparent, becoming
the room, the sofa, the fog, the twittering inside.

It's the love sickness! It's the damned old nausea
of desire, the ague that shakes the last right angle
of reason from your bones
and turns the world to stupid
metaphors for passion.

You peer through the fog like a nearsighted hiker
on a stony seaside path.
Your toes and knees are gone, and the rest of you
dissolving fast: soon you'll be nothing
but the buzz of love, the ache, the fever.

And now, out there, where a window once was,
you think you see the face of the one you love!
It shines toward you like a tiny moon
on a misty night, or a lucky penny,
or a pale expensive sugar candy.

The Cure

1

You go to see the lover, the kind physician, you say,
I'm sick of love.
                    He says
you're a fool, a nuisance, a joke.

You swoon with desire, you beg him to stroke your forehead
with his chill fingers, you offer him your knuckles, your wrists,
your ankles, and all your fingernails.
                                        He declines.
Polite but cold. Explains he's allergic to your skin.
Implies you have a noxious odor.

His icy instruments flash, the chains he fastens to your ribs
are colder than the waters of Lapland, they're made of black iron
dug from the trenches of death.
                                But even as you cringe from them
you smile, you toss your curls like a cheerleader in Houston,
show him your eyelids, invite him
to a picnic in the honeycolored meadow
you found last summer.
                        He says never, he says
forget it, he looks at your bones the way a logger
looks at redwoods: he wants to chop you down, only
he wonders which way you'll fall.

2

So you fall for him, thinking
what a beautiful axe he has, what a shame
to dull that shimmering blade with blood.

Now you're very far down, among stumps and tufts: now
the cure begins, here where the granite banks
cut off the sun and the nettles teach your skin to hate.

A fine dust of dislike rubs through your pores,
your nostrils inhale contempt like swamp gas,
you thrash and grunt in the furious ditch

until the acid takes hold, your blood floods
with the dark brew that collects under stones, rots logs,
lops trees into witchy shapes.

You get on your feet slowly, you're as strong as anyone now,
at last you can stand up for yourself:
you've become a natural marvel, a beautiful pink nettle.

Even your mother would scream
if she touched you.

The Last Poem About
the Snow Queen

Then it was that little Gerda walked into the Palace,
through the great gates, in a biting wind. . . . She saw Kay,
and knew him at once; she flung her arms round his neck,
held him fast, and cried, "Kay, little Kay, have I found you
at last?"
But he sat still, rigid and cold.
—Hans Christian Andersen, "The Snow Queen"

You wanted to know "love" in all its habitats, wanted
to catalog the joints, the parts, the motions, wanted
to be a scientist of romance: you said
you had to study everything, go everywhere,
even here, even
this ice palace in the far north.

You said you were ready, you'd be careful.
Smart girl, you wore two cardigans, a turtleneck,
furlined boots, scarves,
a stocking cap with jinglebells.
And over the ice you came, gay as Santa,
singing and bringing gifts.

Ah, but the journey was long, so much longer
than you'd expected, and the air so thin,
the sky so high and black.
What are these cold needles, what are these shafts of ice,
you wondered on the fourteenth day.
What are those tracks that glitter overhead?

The one you came to see was silent,
he wouldn't say "stars" or "snow,"
wouldn't point south, wouldn't teach survival.

And you'd lost your boots, your furs,
now you were barefoot on the ice floes, fingers blue,
tears freezing and fusing your eyelids.

Now you know: this is the place
where water insists on being ice,
where wind insists on breathlessness,
where the will of the cold is so strong
that even the stone's desire for heat
is driven into the eye of night.

What will you do now, little Gerda?
Kay and the Snow Queen are one, they're a single
pillar of ice, a throne of silence—
and they love you
the way the teeth of winter
love the last red shred of November.

What He Hates / What He Loves

1

You strip away your silky blouse, your
frilly bark, soft armor.
Nude as a peeled tree, you stare
at your pink-white body: swollen,
female, pulpy where it should be rough,
damp where it should be dry,
open where it should be closed. . . .

That's what he hates the most!
More than the mushy breasts, the tender belly,
he hates that swamp inside you,
that moist cleft where flowers quiver,
and darker things, night birds who call from
heavy branches, nests of speckled eggs, small
leaves warm with the weight of the sunset.

Ah, the marsh flesh, the stuff that gushes,
aches, leaks, the stuff
that sighs all night—*What's the matter?*
what's the matter?—how he hates
its muddy longing!
Day after day, now,
you watch him thinning, reddening, hardening:

he's climbing out of the snow of his past,
turning himself into Phaeton, the sunscorched one,
the one who fled the swamp of women

on fiery hooves, through God-rings
buzzing with perpetual light.
You hide in the damp shed at the edge of the swamp, you
call through wreaths of shadow, ripples, silences.

2

He claps a hand on the hand of
the man beside him: hot speech
of bodies sealed up, rough, dry,
instrumental as swords: sword meets
sword. *Son, brother, comrade,
lover,* he says. When you
show him the child's scar, he turns away.

When you tell him about the dead dog,
he says, *Let's change the subject.*
When bird notes pierce the mist
he pats your knee, clears his throat,
puts fast jazz on the stereo.
Phaeton's embers flicker in his eyes.
All around him the sound of hoofbeats, wheels, flame.

Your sweet swamp dries up.
You forget your own name.

You See the Armless Woman

Why are you afraid when you see the armless woman
on some cold suburban corner?
Why do you clasp your own wrists?

The armless woman holds a pen between her teeth,
she types with her toes,
she's competent and springy, wears

a purse like a satin halter around her neck,
smiles, beguiles.
Why do you weep for her invisible knuckles,

why do you shiver
when she flames along the street,
straight as a candle?

Step and step, you follow her,
your feet printing odd words
in yards and puddles:

Give me back that curve of my elbow
where I once hid five diamonds,
give me my wrist where a ruby burned when I was twelve,

let me have back the amber stones of my forearms,
and the joints of my fingers
that once were ivory, amethyst, topaz. . . .

A Year Later

A year later you wonder how you ever loved him.
After all, you tell yourself, he was never more
than a frog, not even pretending to be a prince.
Even then, you think, even in those convulsions of love,
you saw the warts,
the leafslick spots, the cloak of slime:

he was silent because he couldn't speak,
motionless because he couldn't walk.
And yes, you knew it! Yes!
You only loved your own love, only
feasted on your own heart, only cherished
your own fondness for frogs.

But even as you rock and reprimand,
rock and groan, eyes shut in shame,
you remember the forest clearing,
the mossy lip of the well, the way the black water
fell to the center of the stone world,
a shaft of ice that split the grass,

and then there were ripples, circles,
animal honkings—*rivet, rivet*—
and your frog leaped out of silence.
As you sprawled on the lumpy ground, your own
reflection grew in the pool
where he rode like a toy boat.

You bent to kiss the water near him,
wanting to enter his cold glisten,
wanting to seize and wear him like a brooch,

wanting to swallow him as if he were a measure
of some bitter, alien liqueur.
Down and down you bent,

toward the emerald skin, the golden eyes,
closer than ever before
to your own wavering face.

The Return of the Muse

You always knew you wrote for him, you said
He is the father of my art, the one who watches all night,
chainsmoking, never smiling, never satisfied.
You liked him because he was carved from glaciers,
because you had to give him strong wine to make him human,
because he flushed once, like a November sunset,
when you pleased him.

But you didn't love him.
You thought that was part of the bargain.
He'd always be there like a blood relative,
a taciturn uncle or cousin,
if you didn't love him. You'd hand him poems,
he'd inspect them, smoke, sip, a business deal,
and that would be that.

Then he went away and you hardly noticed.
Except you were happy, you danced on the lawn,
swelled like a melon, lay naked long mornings,
brushed your hair more than you needed.
Your breasts grew pink and silky,
you hummed, you sucked the pulp of oranges, you forgot
all about words.

         And when you were
absolutely ignorant,
         he came back,
his jacket of ice flashed white light,
his cap of pallor bent toward you, genteel, unsmiling.
He lit a cigarette, crossed his legs,
told you how clumsy you were.

Ah, then, love seized you like a cramp,
you doubled over in the twist of love.
You shrieked. You gave birth to enormous poems.

He looked embarrassed and said how bad they were.
They became beasts, they grew fangs and beards.
You sent them against him like an army.

He said they were all right
but added that he found you, personally,
unattractive.

   You howled with love,
you spun like a dervish with rage, you
kept on writing.

II

Blood Pressure

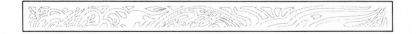

Accident

Something rushes out of the black broth
at the other end of the road, a red needle,
sirens weeping, splotches of light

punching holes in silence.
We slow to a clumsy procession
and shamble hood to hull

past the theater of blood on the dirt shoulder
where pale curved shapes arrange themselves
above flat black ones.

Stretchers, broken glass, a bashed VW—
if we could all get out and tiptoe past
we all would:

I feel the old wound in my eyelid
opening again, the slit
that lets in darkness

and shows me how it took an hour for forty cars
to press the dead deer on yesterday's road
into a dull mat,

the slit of vision
keen as a splinter that goes in and in
and still more deeply in.

Singles, or,
Never Eat Standing Up

It's different with us, she said.
We're singles. Friendship
is all we have.

You have to understand, he said.
I'm a single. My cats
are my family.

It's fantastic, she said.
Since becoming a single I've really
gotten into myself.

Every Friday night we have a hot tub party, he said.
TGIF. BYOB.
Singles Only.

When they come in around six o'clock, she said,
and they only buy yogurt and catfood,
I know they're singles.

I went alone into the country.
At night when the cold pressed against the windows
I pulled down all the shades.

Since you left, he said,
I've been dead inside. It isn't easy
to be a single.

Nowadays most of these condominiums are taken by singles, she said.
They like the Jacuzzi, the sauna, the two swimming pools,
and the yoga classes.

Don't listen to her, she's jealous, he said.
Can't you see she's just another single lady
trying to put the make on me?

Never eat standing up, she said.
Pamper yourself, fix yourself that fancy dinner, make yourself
your own special guest.

We expected something different, he said.
We thought we'd get married. We even
bought life insurance.

Why do you mope around like this, she said.
Why don't you enjoy it while you have it, why don't you live
    like a young modern
or a swinging single?

I went alone into the country.
Every afternoon I walked on the empty road, in the fog,
almost always frightened.

I don't know if I could stand that cruise, she said.
What if they were all retirees? What if there weren't any
eligible singles?

That's a useful column in the *Daily Cal*, he said.
New ways to masturbate, really solid tips on foreplay, especially ideal
for singles.

I went to Paris with my girlfriend, she said.
We sat all day in this little café, but we weren't looking for
    pickups, we were just so glad to be
singles again.

I think it was Margaret Mead, he said,
who said that at fifty every American male should have a new job
and a new lover.

Even after her mastectomy, she let another guy into her house, she
    said.
She gave him the key. She wasn't cut out
to be a single.

I won't tell you his name but it's been great, he said.
I want to live forever! I'm going to come out of the closet, lose
    weight, get a real tan
and buy a rowing machine.

I went alone into the country. I was single.
Every night I drew the shades and sat by the fire
doing my yoga.

Food is one of my main interests, he said.
Kentucky black bean soup is so nummy, and Margaritas, and
    poached salmon, and Brunswick stew.
You think so, too?

Reproduction

April. The hard green seeds
of the Ficus beniamina
suddenly thrust out—arthritic knobs,

little nuts with no kernels of
pleasure in them—
and we ache, we suffer from "spring fever."

Sitting at the round oak table
our friend snaps off one of the tree's fingers:
"He told the marriage counselor

it was no good five years ago,
and I was stunned.
If I'd known he felt that way,

I wouldn't have had a child."

We sip our wine,
and the Ficus droops like a menstruating woman:

its shivery twigs
seem to want to
make some declaration too:

I wished to track the sun in Fiji,
I longed for air and space, why am I
extruding my self in painful pellets?

"I suppose there's still some hope," our
friend observes, "though
the kid's been ruined by her father."

Up the coast, sprayed by fast tides,
do the Bishop pines also suffer?
Their neatly finished, woody cones

lumber upward,
awkward as unclaimed toys,
ridiculously smothered with pollen.

"Of course, she has bonded with me
exclusively," the mother says;
"I am all she has."

Phaeton

For years you've watched them from behind white curtains,
enormous horses with iron hooves, their breath
scrawled across the sky like jet trails, flanks

huge as Adirondacks, manes the tangled brush
where the three-year-old child is lost
and the rabbit screams in the hunter's snare.

Their hides heave and sizzle, their nostrils
are holes from which oblivion pours in wreaths,
their teeth high stalactites of dry ice.

A spindly kid, blond, uncertain, you hang on
to your mother's middle finger where
the emerald ring winks like spring,

don't talk much, play mostly with girls:
other boys ignore you; your father's
been away for years, fighting overseas.

They're your father's horses, your mother says,
sultry evenings when the great hooves
tattoo the stone stable floor.

*Don't be frightened, they're
your father's horses.* Sometimes
you sneak to the glowing doorway

and stare, stare.
                    Their whinny
pierces you like the shout of light

you saw once when the dawn sun
leaped out of the Atlantic.
You clench small fists.

            You want to
whip those haunches till blood
spurts like a hot lather, a halo;

you want to rip out those stiffened manes
the way a gardener
uproots furious platoons of goldenrod.

Blood Pressure

The white-sleeved woman wraps a rubber
sleeve around your arm, steps back, listens,
whistles.

How it pounds in you, how it
urges through you, how it asserts
its power like a tide of electrons

flashing through your veins, shocking your fingertips,
exhausting the iron gates of your heart.
Alive, always alive, it hisses,

crackling like the lightning snake that splits
the sky at evening, *alive,* a black rain
lashing the hollows of your body,

alive, alive.
You sit quietly on the cold table,
the good boy grown up into

the good man. You say
you want nothing, you'll diet, you
won't complain. Anyway, you say,

you dream of January weather,
hushed and white, the cries of light
silenced by a shield of ice.

Behind your eyes, something
like a serpent moves, an acid tongue
flicking at your cheekbones, something

voracious, whipping your whole body
hard: you're sad, you flush a
dangerous pink, you tell her

you can't understand the fierce rain
inside you, you've always hated that awful
crackling in your veins.

To a Man Who Advises Maturity

Only October but already you dream of resignation,
already you shovel snow in your head
and wear maturity like a winter suit—
severe cut, expensive wool, handsewn buttonholes.

Renunciation, you advise, is good
for women and poets: it purifies
the blood, blots out adjectives, modulates
that high shrill female voice.

You make me want to scream, make me
want to fly around your head in circles,
fat and shrill as a summer gull,
and shriek in a voice that splits your seams:

Your maturity has lead feathers!
Look! Frost is growing like mold
in your armpits, and behind your eyelids
a winter twilight thickens.

I want to wake you up with a slap and get you
gasping like a baby, I want to make
a blood-orange October morning
happen outside your window

as if it were your own
bright idea.

Belgian Endive:
For an Old Friend

You say you want me to write this poem about your favorite salad as if you were asking me for a password that would carry both of us across some invisible frontier. You point to the white leaves and tell me how they are kept colorless, how green is forbidden them, how the refusal of sun makes them bitter.

My ruby flashes. In the blood-light of my mind I see the stone farmhouse in the lowlands, the brown plain reaching toward the sea, the trees whose branches slope and droop, the Flemish wife with her lips set in a thin line.

Beneath her kitchen is a cellar where the endives grow in their dark garden. Morning and night she visits them, wiping her hands on her apron, thinning and trimming, remote as a surgeon. Above them bleak shutters clamp like teeth, spiders spin among black beams.

Here the endives grow into their bloom of bitterness. The Flemish wife leans over the furrow, the breath of the cellar stirs, the endives clench their leaves and urge themselves out of the dirt like small pale phalluses. Wind beats at the farmhouse where those white shapes are rising, rain washes over its slate roof.

I think you already know all this. I think you have seen this place before. Why do you want me to tell you the whole story again?

This Is Not...

This is not the poem you want me to write, not
the poem in which I tell you
how the gold got into your body, how
the hair on your arms became pale and valuable,
how your face changed in the phases of the moon,
glowed, sharpened, cut through clouds.

This is not the poem in which I ask you
to admire the way blue veins map my right breast
like lightning, not the poem
where our bodies lean into each other
like cypresses or rose bushes.

In this poem we go on our journey.
It's late afternoon, late autumn,
bleak and sweet: we drive through a gray drizzle
on shiny dangerous roads.
                          We say
we're going to the coast, we're going
to gather bay leaves, wild grasses, branches of eucalyptus
on the ridge near the sea;
                          we say
we won't be gone long.

At twilight we come to the old inn
on the hillside: it's getting cold,
we stop for wine, notice
the dead leaves blowing around the garden
behind the bar.
                    I'm tired
and vain: I go upstairs

to wash and brush. (I think
I should have some new perfume for you,
something no one has invented yet.)

When I come down
I see you waiting for me
on the stony path among the cold laurels
and the dead blackberries.
                              In this poem
you are only yourself,
and you wait for me—
silent, motionless, a little bored—
in the November garden.

Thinking About an Old Friend

Once, although I guess you're more than six feet
tall and pretty hefty,
I dreamed you were a tiny perfect tree

surrounded by glossy palings
and a sign that said *Noli Me Tangere*
in bristling calligraphy.

No, we aren't (as someone said the other day)
like brother and sister. More like
two only children left alone

in a damp sandbox
with a cracked pail, a broken shovel.
We sit in opposite corners and stare,

wondering what next.
Maybe it would help if we took off these heavy
bodies. Maybe we'd speak more freely.

We could get into the air
and be two breezes, meeting
in silent puffs; we could

become two fistfuls of foam,
hissing hasty messages;
two minor earthquakes, barely perceptible

but deeply mutual.
    Listen,
I bet you'd tell me more

if you were a root and I a stone.
And if we were two splintery boards in
an old farmhouse on the coast of Maine

we'd always have known the whole
length and weight of each other.
We'd lean together all day,

gazing out at the tragically
separate freighters on their random
roads.

In December the winds from Canada
would beat us like black paddles.
Together our bodies would creak and groan,

our only language: we'd know
each other so absolutely
there really would be nothing else to say.

Talking to an Old Friend

My words litter the table like tornup napkins
or lumps of meat that made you sick,
you had to spit them out. You think
even the thought of talk is a transgression,
an embarrassment.
                          I keep on
pouring wine, passing sugar, offering
bread and poems. No. You decline.
Love discomfits you, tears
are too salty, flesh too sour.

I gum a smile over my lips
like a big bandaid. I say,
here's another pat of butter, here's
another poem, another
basket of wishes.
                          Sorry,
you say, *so sorry. . . .*

I stare at my fingers. The black
formica table blurs, boards
below glossy shadows crack
and give way. Underneath
there's something darker than black,
something spinning and churning
like the air that roars between
this peak and that one.
                          Now I know
why mountain climbers don't look down.
Near me the rock slide's beginning—
a sigh of gravel, a few pebbles

leaping out from the cliff face, then
the granite tearing like paper, the easy
casual descent of trees, the wind, the calamity.

I look up fast, trying to find your eyes
that are winking and blue behind
panes of glass. Sunlight
glints on ice. I'm very still. I promise
I'll be very still. You say,
I liked that other silence better.

Sauna

Alone in the sauna, nearsighted, heating up
after a long cold swim alone, I don't
really notice her when she comes in—
a twist of white in the half light, then
a female blur spread flat on the upper bench.
I sit crosslegged, stare at nothing, breathe,
sweat, meditate. And then her voice:
What's wrong? Is something wrong? Or is it just
the heat? I hadn't thought I looked like that:
drenched, exhausted, drippy as Phaedra on
the scorching boards. Naked I swam away
from you, back to my life through a tank of snow.
    But now I'm happy, tingly, in great shape.
    Whose are these sighs? Why does my body weep?

"But I Don't Love Him"

—FOR D.

Thirty thousand feet up, the plane climbing past clouds,
I suddenly see
your great clarity.

The other night we streamed along the freeway;
Silicon Valley to San Francisco to Berkeley,
we were alone with the hum

of your Rabbit's motor,
and you spoke:
"I had to go back to him, I needed a partner. . . .

But I don't love him anymore.
I loved him so much once,
but now no more. . . ."

Thirty thousand feet up, the high sky
is cold as your words. I order extra wine,
smoke, scribble in the flyleaf

of a book called *Classical Greece*.
Next to me a New York couple
debate the virtues of traveling first class,

Matt Dillon gallops on the screen,
The Oresteia staggers grandly
toward catastrophe.

Outside, that transcendent pallor,
a blue I know would kill me.
Even now, the panes are freezing:

if I were draped against the plane,
clinging to the window,
the ice that sealed my fingertips

to 747 plastic
would hold me up.
O Clytemnestra,

why are you so honest, how
are you so clear, so true?
When I hear you say

"I don't love him,"
I pass through the window
into ancient cold,

and I want to find out what love is.
You bend toward me, frosty hair and fingers.
The car rushes forward, the plane hisses.

It says on this page
"Dance for the dearest, the bringer of peace,
Deathless Aphrodite."

O Aphrodite,
I want to learn
what you bring, want to know

why that blue freezes me.

III

The Summer Kitchen

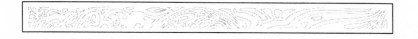

"Empty Nest"

Dream after dream, you go back to the old house.
Your intelligent feet, your fingertips whorled with thought
like the brilliant skin of the blind

lead you down the halls
into rooms where once
you were possible—

       the pantry
where you wept among canisters of whispering flour,
the bedroom whose walls crawled with roses,

the library where you had everything
and nothing to read, the nursery
full of enigmatic shouts. . . .

Your grandmother is in the garden, her cane
guides her past the mint, the phlox, the day lilies,
to the table where your mother and her sister

sit under a pink umbrella, sipping
long sweet drinks, arguing, laughing.
A breeze rises, the June roses sway

and flutter their colors: your dead father
is around the corner, on the porch
snapping pictures of your children.

The house has just been painted:
it's green and white, white and gold,
blue and tan, green and—

What is this cold place, this moment
you've fallen into?
Trapped in its transparency, you

stare at lost shapes
like a mammoth gazing in wonder
at what is still alive.

In the old house
the changeling children leap and glow.
Shivering, you hold out your arms.

Nothing relinquishes you.

In the Golden *Sala*

Sun of Sicilian hillsides,
heat of poppies opening like fierce
boutonnières of Apollo,
light of Agrigento, fretting the sea and the seaside cliffs—
light of the golden *sala*,
the great *sala* of the ruined *palazzo*
where my Sicilian grandmother and her nine children
camped outside Palermo.

Gold leaf, gold moldings,
shredding tapestries with gold threads.
"Once it belonged to a prince.
Mama kept chickens on the terrace
but they came in sometimes, and the donkey too."
Gold chairs, gilt around the windows,
angels with shining hair and empty eyes
staring from the ceiling.

"Mama made our beds in the corners:
the big room scared us, we thought
the prince's ghost was there."
Gold railings where her laundry hung,
gold curtains, new eggs under them.
Her cooking fire in a corner,
the center of the *sala* a cave of gold
for spankings and scoldings.

"Mama was a midwife, knew
everything about herbs and births.
The peasant women came from farms around Palermo
so she could help them."

On floors still streaked with gold
she made them spaces
in the dazzling spaces where the prince once walked.
Gold of forgotten dances, tattered rugs.

When a new baby slid out in a splash of water
he must have looked up, dazed,
toward the prince's Apollonian light,
and the black eyes of the midwife
and the black eyes of the midwife's nine blackhaired children
would have looked quizzically down,
as if from a high cliff by the sea
hot and yellow with new poppies.

The Summer Kitchen

In June when the Brooklyn garden
boiled with blossom,
when leaflets of basil lined the paths
and new green fruitless fingers of vine
climbed the airy arbor roof,

my Sicilian aunts withdrew
to the summer kitchen,
the white bare secret room
at the bottom of the house.
Outside, in the upper world,

sun blistered the bricks of the tiny
imitation-Taormina terrace where fierce
socialisti uncles
chainsmoked Camels and plotted politics;
nieces and nephews tusseled

among thorny bloodcolored
American roses;
a pimply concrete
birdbath-fountain dribbled ineffectual
water warm as olive oil.

Cool and below it all,
my aunts labored among great cauldrons
in the spicy air
of the summer kitchen: in one kettle
tomatoes bloomed into sauce;

in another, ivory *pasta*
leaped and swam;
on the clean white table
at the center of the room
heads of lettuce flung themselves open,

and black-green poles of zucchini
fell into slices of yellow
like fairytale money.
Skidding around the white
sink in one corner

the trout that Uncle Christopher brought back
from the Adirondacks gave up
the glitter of its fins
to the glitter of *Zia* Francesca's
powerful knife.

Every August day *Zia* Petrina
rose at four to tend the morning:
smoky Greek chignon
drawn sleek,
she stood at the sink.

Her quick shears
flashed in the silence,
separating day from night, trunk
from branch, leaf
from shadow.

As the damp
New World sunrays struggled to rise
past sooty housetops,
she'd look suddenly up
with eyes black as the grapes

that fattened in the arbor:
through one dirt-streaked window
high above her
she could see the ledge of soil
where her pansies and geraniums anchored.

Higher still,
in tangles of heat,
my uncles' simmering garden grew,
like green steam swelling from the cool
root of her kitchen.

Beets

You disguise yourselves as dark-skinned stones,
plumed in purple and green,
but perhaps you're really an army,
filing toward summer, crusaders
for sweetness and heat,
                              or perhaps

a caravan of Russian traders,
modestly shrunken but bearing
goods of great value—a cargo
of rubies, for instance
and little magic sacks of blood. . . .

Dwarf heads, tiny warriors
rocking silently across the fields,
I know you know some secret!

Dry cold days when the ground is hard
you stick to your positions,
as if to say: *Context is all, order, origins.*
Pull me from my place in line
and I am lost!

But when the earth is wet and easy
you let go like drunken Cossacks,
as if murmuring, *Ah, pleasure*
of surrender, O happy nights
alone in the tavern, under the moon!

In long-ago Russia my twelve-year-old grandma,
the *shabbas goy,* knelt in the black thick furrows

of the summer steppe and plucked up
baskets and baskets of fat-cheeked beets.
Every night her peasant grandmother stewed them
and married them to sour cream, onions, cabbages.

When the long winter struck the tundra with iron,
they remembered that ritual meal, remembered—
as they sighed beside the great black Russian stove
and the samovar hissed and they scooped out
coals for the Jews next door—

that you were still marching somewhere,
that there was still a secret
procession of blood,
                    under the ground.

Grandpa

Garlic and cigars recall you, stuffed mushrooms,
spinach ravioli, Genoa haunting your kitchen,

and you with your dragging foot—
bad circulation, maybe a stroke—

5'3", bald, gray forehead, gray mustache, failed
restaurateur, failed painter, thinning as you cooked,

thinning to the one you were in the bottle-green
Hotel Negresco uniform in Nice,

only now in Queens, pining for the old farm,
the hills above the sea. . . .

When they paced the cobbled wharf at Genoa
planning their moves five centuries ago,

what did they imagine? The men
must have been seamen: leaning landward like old walls,

they must have dreamed you as a wave
breaking on some far island. You must

have been their intention for the future. When the great
ship set sail, heeling and running free,

you lay in the hold, naked of uniforms,
painter of frescoes, master of promised spices,

rosy, perfect. What accident
of the mid-Atlantic

turned you into a scrap of cargo
lost by the civilization of the wind—

the calm sea, the prosperous voyage—
that left you and your dragging foot behind?

The Twelve Dancing Princesses

1

Why am I distracted all day, dreaming of the twelve princesses, their heavy satin skirts, their swift flight across dark fields, their slow cold sensual descent into the lake? All day the twelve princesses circle my furniture like gulls, crying out in a strange language, proposing mysterious patterns with their wings. Below them indecipherable ripples wash over the carpet like white lies.

At midnight the gates of the lake swing wide: the princesses enter the halls of water. In that blue-green ballroom they dance like minnows, darting among stones, leaping away from circles of light. Even as I write these words, each solitary dancer is spinning in the palace of shadow, spinning through night so deep that the call of the owl is not heard, and the twelve underground princes, wrapped in sleep, row silently away across the lake.

2

I am the scholar of the dark armchair—the crimson wingchair of 1945, the overstuffed gold-tufted armchair of 1948, the downy satin chair of 1952, and always the dark chair beneath, the chair immense as the lap of a grandfather, the chair in which I sit reading the tale of the twelve dancing princesses.

Winter. Wind on the fire escape. The hush of snow. Summer. Shouts in the street. Horns, bells, processions of cars. I curl myself into the dark armchair. I shape my body to its shape, I do not lift my eyes.

Miles away, at the edge of the city, the twelve princesses flee toward the airfield. Night swells the arms of the chair that holds me. The princesses dance in the sky like helicopters. Below them the lights of the runway burn in silence, serious as lines on a map or instructions in a secret book: severe frontiers, all crossing forbidden.

Hooked Rug

I was eight. I stared at the gray hooked rug,
its pattern of pink timidity—a rabbit
twisting through a pale forest,
pious birds overhead.

I stared and stared. Why
was the rabbit running, what was the bad fact
somebody's hook
had knotted into that center?

I stared. I thought I'd be sick.
From the kitchen leaked the voices
of my parents, brooding on dinner.
I was eight. What did I know

besides sweating at ballet, that clumsy
jeté into the mirror,
and trembling at punchball, the cold
schoolyard with its loops and lines?

I was eight. I toed
the line. I stared at the rabbit.
She leaped under the birds but
they swooped nowhere,

they started no cry, they were
only threads, and she was
only a lump of wool:
she was fixed in the rug, her pink

flight from the dark border
was stopped, and stayed in place
like the bedroom wall,
like the boards on the floor.

Jackson Heights
Apartment Kitchen, 1948

Yellow paint thick as buttercream
glosses the cupboards of the tiny Queens
apartment kitchen; yellow
linoleum on the floor, bland as
the landlord's jaundiced look.
In winter, we open the narrow window
a crack. Smoke from broiling chops
curls out like dragon's breath.
At six o'clock, my father the ex-altarboy
stands, glass in hand, in the jolly doorway.
In nomine patris, he says,
lowering his chef's apron over his head.
　　The walls lean toward him
　　kindly as slices of Wonder Bread.

New Year's Eve

I was just eleven, the War was over,
and my aunt's big Williamsburg kitchen
glowed like those great old-country hearths
I read about in fairy tales.
                            A block away
the Bushwick Avenue El
thundered through snowclouds, its Cyclops
forehead piercing unimaginable Brooklyn distances. . . .

New Year's Eve! My parents danced
at the Forest Hills Inn in Queens
while my Aunt Francesca babysat
me and her lasagna sauce.
                            Sullen, American,
almost plump enough to need "Chubbettes,"
I watched my teen-age cousins samba
with "men in their twenties."

My cousins were studying Spanish and wore Carmen Miranda
dresses: their ruffles leaping like windblown leaves, my cousins
did mysterious hops and skips, swaying to South American rattles:
my cousins sang Argentinian songs in their Americanized
Italian opera voices. . . .
                            At midnight
a tall man pulled beautiful Virginia
into a corner

and kissed her, like Cary Grant
kissing Rosalind Russell. Outside
snowflakes sugared the leafless
twigs on Uncle Frank's grape arbor

and the two-dollar florist's Xmas wreath
on the front door. When no one was looking
I stole a scrap of the wreath and scotch-
taped it into my "Journal of Thoughts and Events."

Underneath I printed
"In memory of New Year's Eve 1948,
A New Year's Eve I shall never forget."

Easter 1949

The eggs glowed on the table. Ovals, colors.
It was April. Pale sky, thin leaves, bare stones.
We sat in grandma's plush and leather chairs.
They had high curlicued backs, like thrones.
We ate lamb, asparagus, quivering mint jelly,
first strawberries—sweet and bright and fat.
Watched a dozen eggs shimmer faintly
in the center of a bone-white plate.
I was twelve. Bored. The women argued.
What did Picasso *mean* demanded my Catholic
aunt. What did *Jesus* mean my agnostic
mother cried. Next door my father snored.
  The eggs glowed on the table, oiled, dyed.
  Inside each one something cold and hard.

Pinocchio

1

Eyes on a slab of wood,
Giapetto's gaze,

as if through all those obstinate
layers, grainy veils,

film on film of forest, spring, fall,
root, bole, burl,

Pinocchio's wide round painted eyes
met his eyes.

2

Boys romp in the roadway. Pinocchio
romps and clatters. Overhead
April rattles twigs of chestnut,
cypress, pine. When Pinocchio

looks at the forest does he see
the eyes of cousins. Does he dream
a tickle of moss
on his painted scalp?

He creaks in his sleep!

3

Ill wood, ill wind, all nose
for sniffing out what's done, what's dung,

Pinocchio drifts in the jaws of winter,
fish or father, whale or wave:

everything's black down here,
nothing to touch except

the teeth of water.
This is the world, digesting

him, he thinks. Soon he'll be
a stump, a plank, driftwood, deadwood,

then a skin of paper, then a word,
a *what.* . . . And why?

What was "the truth" anyway?

4
A field. A hut. A hearth.
An iron grate. Flames, ashes.

Crows clack in the field, their gullets
open and close, ancient gates.

In the hearth ashes toss and shift,
flames mutter, wooden shapes spatter,

simmer: their sap gasps
bleak phrases: *Lies, all lies.*

Noses are lies. Breath.
Fathers. Forests.

Are lies. There is no.
"Truth." Anyway.

5

Giapetto walks on the hillside
in the evening cool, paces
leafy tunnels, admires
sighing lanes, muses, sees
a hillside full of boys
disguised as trees.

Jump Rope

In front of the imitation-palace apartment house,
beyond the shadows of the lobby
where the gilt-edged doorman dreams and smokes,

the skip rope,
whipping like the sea,
lives between the wrists of two grave girls,

Its one-hand-clapping steady scrape and snap
speaks in a rhythm that seems to come
from some invisible whale's belly:

Enter my magic peristalsis and be changed.
Enter and skip!
Enter and dance!

Enter the grown-up pulsing
house of the rope,
and jump,

jump for your life!

Jackson Heights

Red brick, gold brick, trim colonial white,
the apartment palaces rose for miles along
the shady avenues of Jackson Heights,
their hedges firm, their names a WASP song,
the Colton, the Buckingham, the Iveagh Leaf,
their lobbies stage-sets of gentility,
sofas and chairs a little larger than life
as if arranged for a giant tea party.
At fifteen, I knew this was "making it."
Each day, "Thank God for Queens," my mother said.
Sicily was what she tried to forget—
the stony village, the farmyard, the donkey shit.
   Then why did my Spanish boyfriend kiss my ear
   and murmur sexily "How can *you* live here?"

For Edna St. Vincent Millay

Caught in Arnold Genthe's net of petals,
you muse in the Museum of Modern Art, not
understanding the shards of the avant garde—
the Cubist nude you thought just "piles of shingles,"
the blank triangles, the twisted metals
not meant, anyway, to pierce *your* heart.
Were you only the smart kid from Maine
you claimed you were? Were you, poetess,
no more than chalice for the sickly wine
that makes your younger sisters gag and curse?
"It Girl of '22," your dead renown
billows around you like a faded dress—
    but once we loved you: reading all night long,
    we hadn't learned that you (and we) were wrong.

Rissem

I was sixteen, a freshman, a former Catholic Buddhist,
a sonnet-writer, no longer overweight but more than ever
ambitious for romance. At night in my lumpy dorm bed
I counted the number of would-be "lovers" I had,
sometimes adding the names of even my mildest fans
to fatten the list.

                    You were twenty.
Your forehead was too high, your IQ (you said) one hundred eighty,
and I called my mother in Queens to tell her about you.
You'd already had mono and worried about potency!
You had loved many brilliant girls in Brooklyn!
But none like me.

We put our initials together—your R.I.S., my S.E.M.—and became
    rissem.
We collected Tagliavini records for the high Cs.
We stole steaks from the IGA.
We gave your English bicycle a name I've forgotten.
We kissed on campus in front of the coeds and statues.
People thought we were disgusting.

But when you came to my archery class
on the windy hillside beyond the dormitories,
you always made bullseyes,
even when the wind was strongest.
One night I cried all night in a narrow rooming-house bed,
wedged between you and the wall:

I saw the truth: the day would come
when I'd be twenty-eight, you'd be thirty-two,

we'd be married to other lovers, have other names.
And you were going to invent a solar battery!
You were going to discover the truth about aging
and perhaps prevent death!

When you died, fifteen years and three marriages
after we'd said goodbye on the Fifty-ninth Street station,
your best friend told me the driver of your hearse got lost
on the Brooklyn-Queens Expressway.
It was incredible, he said. *He would have loved it.*
He would have thought it was a great scene!

Sometimes I like to think we are still *rissem,*
a slender ageless androgyne from another planet.
With bow and arrow we hunt among strange craters.
Breathlessness doesn't bother us, or weightlessness.
The list of our lovers is long but we are indifferent
to all of them. On our planet

we bicycle faster than the speed of light.
In our extragalactic language
there are no words for "love" or "death."

Invocation

After you were dead a year,
I was still meeting you everywhere.
That time in the garden,
I glanced past my three-year-old son

and there you were by the chain-link fence.
My brooding prince!—
you wore your old look
of sulky independence.

I wanted to say "You can't come back,
you can't haunt a garden,
a street, a house
you never lived in!"

It was almost Easter,
a few tulips, chancy weather,
and my little boy
dug among the wavery

stalks of hopeful daisies,
tremulous day lilies.
I thought you stared like Byron,
thought you wanted to rage like Satan

at his small pail,
his glittering shovel. . . .
and now, twenty years later,
again it's Easter,

and again
the only resurrection
lifts new day lilies
into an indifferent breeze.

Old friend, dead one,
I will pour you a glass of wine,
I will stain
a white cloth with my libation.

Come back again,
come to the edge of the garden
and look into the flesh and bone
of this house where you can't come in.

For Miss Lewis
and Miss Newton

As you walked through the streets of Vienna—already a grey-beard and weighed down by all the cares of family life—you might come unexpectedly on some well-preserved elderly gentleman, and would greet him humbly almost because you had recognized him as one of your former schoolmasters. But afterwards, you would stop and reflect "Was that really he? or only someone deceptively like him? How youthful he looks! And how old you yourself have grown. . . ." These men became our substitute fathers. That was why, even though they were still quite young, they struck us as so mature and so unattainably adult.

—Sigmund Freud

And our mothers: what it meant
to love them, to want to be loved
by them—those anonymous phone calls we made
just to hear them say "hello? hello?";

those afternoons we lurked a foot or two
beyond the classroom door
and, looking in, we saw them, beautiful, absorbed,
grading papers at the scratched oak desk!

Allie Lewis: Lexington Avenue, Central Park,
wherever I walked
I carried you in my head,
your halo of black hair, tender eyes. . . .

Cornelia Newton: on Bleecker Street, Macdougal Street,
you haunted me,
your shabby leopard coat, wispy voice,
gray-blonde ringlets. . . .

How youthful you look now,
and how old I've grown!
Adult as a briefcase, I'm carried
over the Rockies by TWA.

Lines of snow
loop below me,
hieroglyphs in a white script
that's called maturity.

Enormous trees shadow the dark trails
on the lost half of the cliff.
What's behind me now
was ahead of you then.

Yet your faces, traced in the *massif,*
still stare, stare up at me,
your high cheekbones glimmer,
your hair—yellow, black, gray—

changes its colors with the seasons.

Low Tide

Dissatisfaction of my youth, pigtailed eight-year-old
poet of Jackson Heights, I know
you're somewhere still, still keeping house
under the sea, under the bitter waters.

Low tide. I pick my way among the pilings
down the long rotting pier
to the ocean beds where you huddle
among slippery stones.

I'll find you, I'll pluck you out
though the claws of silence
skin my fingers
and my knuckles turn to salt.

You're there!—
practicing on the dreary mahogany spinet
where new white thin-shelled mussels
cling together for comfort.

Over and over, dutiful and stupid,
you play those scales, the key of F, the key of G,
as if in such numbers there was safety.
And under an awning of seaweed

you dawdle over your shoelaces,
staring down at the frayed gray bedroom rug
where the rabbit runs away forever,
away into some invisible forest. . . .

You're there—ten, twelve, fourteen, sixteen—
there with your "sorrows"
and your untouched geometry books,
where the brackish water laps.

I am the piano teacher who never finished the lesson,
I am the mother who taught you *plus* and *minus*,
the father who cried "It's never too late!"
the grandma who mended seams and quarrels,

the boyfriend who dreamed of murder.
Even now,
as you drift through the tidepools in pleated skirt
and knee socks, writing clumsy poems,

I'm groping my way toward you,
down the long pier,
in the sea fog,
among the screaming gulls.

My Grandmother in Paris

Paris. 1900. A sky of corrugated iron. Snow and mud.
Beggars like heaps of debris on street corners.
Women with pink cheeks melting in doorways.
Splashes of laughter, church bells, creaking boots.
Puccini's Paris, Paris of *La Bohème,* Paris
of garrets and prisons, Paris of sweet fevers, Paris

of phlegm and sweat, ivory breasts, skylights, *opéra:*
Paris of Wagner and Rilke, Paris of delicious
nineteenth-century melancholy, Paris where streetlights
glisten through the winter twilight
like pomegranates in hell.
                              Twilight.

My grandmother walks in the Bois de Boulogne
under frosted chestnuts. She's twelve years old,
a roundfaced girl just come from Russia,
her hair in skinny braids
like strange embroidery around her head.
She's on her way to the house of the Russian priest

where her mother cooks and cleans
but she watches, wondering, as carriages plunge
through the slush of the Bois, their lamps
leaping like goblin heads, their blanketed horses
clopping docile as cows through all the Paris noise.
Baudelaire is dead, Rimbaud dead in Africa, Gertrude Stein

thinking in Baltimore, Picasso painting in Barcelona.
My grandmother has learned three words of French:
allo, comment, combien. Amedée, the boy she's

going to marry four years from now
is in Nice with his sister Eugénie,
who will die next year at nineteen,

and his sister Rosette, who will die at forty.
My grandmother is still tired from last week.
She stops to sit on a low wall beside the road
and begins to shape a tiny angel out of crumbs of snow.
From a passing *fiacre* a young clerk off to the *opéra*
sees her round pink face suspended like a small balloon

in the blue air.
                    What is she thinking
as she pats a cold celestial head and frozen wings?
Is she remembering the awful trainride
across Europe, the bonfires at the Polish border, the shouts
as the engine chuffed into Berlin? No. She rises,

makes her angel into a snowball and tosses it at a tree.
She's thinking of Russia, of her grandmother back in the room
in Rostov-on-the-Don, of the ice like silver on the river
all winter and long into spring, of the black fields
outside town and the old stories of Baba Yaga and the tales
she has also heard of the redhaired cossack

said to be her own father.
                    She walks faster.
It's late and cold. Her mother will worry.
The fat priest will be cross. Paris
grows around her like an enigmatic alphabet.
Even the trees are different here. No firs, no birches!

As she walks, Baba Yaga's house on chicken legs
steps delicately away across snowy meadows
and her father the cossack, with his furry animal head, fierce teeth,
                                        red beard,
gallops into glacial distances.
(Does she suspect that from now on
she'll never really know any language again?)

Tomorrow the priest will be sixty. To celebrate
he'll buy a Swiss cane at the Galéries Lafayette.
                                        In seventy years
my grandmother will twirl that cane and dance a twostep
among the eucalyptuses above San Francisco Bay,
singing me the song about the lost princess of the Volga

while, far below, the cold Pacific
glitters like an ice field.

IV
The Parachutist's
Wife

The Three Sisters

1 The One Who Went Away

They said she "thought about it for a long time."
What to do. How. After all, they said,
she felt she was no longer herself,
she was a smile printed on a pillow,
a web of thread,
a dead skin of linen.

So she went. Past the secret keyhole,
through the waist-high door, into the tower room
where it's always spring, the windows are thick as bricks
to keep out the cold, the floor is sweet with rushes,
the bed a heap of fragrant boughs,
the tiny hearth burns silver coals all night.

Now all night
they cruise around her tower in the old VW bus,
lights out, a dark weight
crushing the grassy path around the tower, pulling
at the great stones like the drag of blood
against unknown hollows of the body.

She smiles in the dark. Sniffs April colors.
Her hearth is the eye of a lilac! Her bed's a jonquil!
Still the bus creaks by with its ponderous tread,
the husband with wide strained eyes doubled over the wheel
as if it were some inexplicable shame,
the tangled feuding kids, the seatbelts, the tennis rackets. . . .

Candied violets, gulls' feathers, sugar biscuits:
clear as air, light waters
ripple over the stones of her mind.
All night the thin voices of her daughters
swirl around her window
like forgotten flakes of snow.

2 The One Who Stayed Behind

In her right hand she holds the moon,
that lamp of milk.
Out of her left, stars spill, white seeds
from a pod of light.
Behind her the wise
staircase rises, always rises.
Yet still she holds to her level,
she's calm, doesn't smile.

Her yard spreads around her like a clean napkin
lit by milk, her daughters
spin through fat bushes like tops, her sons
somersault among thistles.
She's calm, doesn't smile.
But a blue scar crosses her left breast, she winces,
and you know: she's the one
who married the frost king,

the little girl they sent in high fur boots to the far north,
the one who swallowed the needle of ice, who's chained
by vow and virtue
to the unchanging ruler of snow
with his frost-pale hair and his eyes that are
magic as the blue wounds
that split the glaciers at sundown.
She's the one!

Her dishes shatter in her kitchen,
her children tumble and shriek, her human
husband twists in the ache of life.
She's calm, doesn't smile.
The ice inside her rivets her
into the stone of earth and moon,
the pure rock at the center of everyone.
She looks away.

Ah, there,
where the staircase coils up and up,
a single moth is flying,
a small gray puff of wind
like a fleck of dust in a jar of milk,
or a drift of shadow
on the still stone
face of the moon.

3 The Third Sister

She's the one who lives on the hem of the meadow,
the sandy edge of solitude where the cliff
dips a few tentative stones toward the sea.

Her seasons are early spring and late fall,
when the winds rise and the weird
transformations begin:

where she steps
jets of green light lift and die on the gray
face of the weather,

and her children say,
Now she's deciding, now things will settle.
But they never do, for she's

the border-breaker, the restless one, the one
who sits all night sketching the dark
and sleeps all day with sunlight scorching her eyelids.

The man who loves her knows
she'll never make up her mind, her mind's
a rumpled bed where she lies with him long afternoons,

half naked, half slippery satin,
half embracing, half
turning away.

Outside the quaking house
her laundry flails in the seawind
like flags of truce or banners signaling for help,

as if she were calling on something
at a further, invisible edge, a wind
that might blow another way, a sea

that might be a different color,
a new kind of stone,
or a new season.

Five Potatoes

Heavy and blind, swollen with themselves, five potatoes wobble on the drainboard near the sink. When I met them they were passionate: stitched into thick loam, they drove all their strength into a hundred eyes. Now they've lost their purpose. But anyway I'll peel them, boil them, slice them, feed my children their forgotten visions.

I hum a little under my breath as I scrub and scrape. *Changes,* I sing, *transformations!* The cold water from the tap foams over my fingers. Just now, in Africa, a !Kung grandmother rises, picks up her stick, slings her pack across her shoulder, and walks away from the cooking fire. She's going to ford the river at the narrow place where the trout jump and the leopard comes down to drink, going to travel up the muddy path along the bank in the buzzing early morning light, and dig for yams for her children in the wild field beyond the village.

The Parachutist's Wife

—FOR M. L.

1

Six men turned to smoke in the next square
of air, their plane became wind.
You were twenty-three. Hands over your ears, a roaring
in your veins, a silence
on the radio.

    Flak
knocked twice at the cockpit,
dull knuckles, thumping:
Let me in,
    let me in.

You knew you had to
give yourself to the sky the way we
give ourselves to music—no knowing
the end of the next bar, no figuring
how the chord will fall.

2

The clouds were cold, the plane trembled.
You pulled the cord and the chute
"bloomed like God's love," a heavenly
jockstrap anchoring you in air.

You were happy, you say, you were
never happier than that day, falling
into birth: the archaic
blue-green map of Europe glowed below you.

You were going to camp, you were
going to be free of death.
The pull of the harness, the swaying,
the ropes creaking—it was so peaceful up there,

like a page of Greek or
an afternoon in a Zen monastery
or a long slow stroll around
somebody's grandfather's garden.

3
I'm quiet in my kitchen, I won't
bail out, I don't think it would be the same
for me, I think if I

fell like that the hands of flak
would strip me as I
swung from the finger of God, I'd

offer myself as a bright idea
and a chorus of guns
would stammer holes in my story, nothing

would lift me over the black fangs
of the Alps, I'd dangle
like bait and the savage

map of Europe would eat me up.
I stick like grease to my oven, I wear
a necklace of dust,

my feet root in green stone.
You've forgotten I'm here!
But every morning

there are crystals of ice in my hair
and a winter distance glitters
in the centers of my eyes.

I don't need to stroll through the sky
like a hero:
in my bone cave

I marry the wind.

Twilight

Twilight. Twolight. Light
cut in half by absence, light
dividing itself.

The invisible moves closer, a great
wagon creaking over the treetops.
I let go your hand,

we whisper goodbye, we
divide,
we make way for the phantom wheels.

Late Beethoven

1

Beethoven dozes in a stone courtyard,
solemn head tipped backward, closed eyes
gazing at granite:

behind his lids
minuets of death,
without shapes, without dancers.

The sweetness of that desolation!
Iced feathers, damp ferns
in a slow wind, quartz pebbles

falling one by one
into the black pond at the far
end of the meadow. . . .

2

It's midnight when we come to
the stone house in the pine forest.
Your key enters the lock like a word
that brings meaning to a blind sentence.

No electricity. No moon.
You click your flashlight on
and walk three times around the room,
splashing light across locked cupboards.

Yes, there's Beethoven
asleep on a couch against the wall.
His snores and wishes fill the air
like the breathless drone of a fan

or like the white breath of water
hurrying over cold stones.

3
For a moment Beethoven
is half or more than half

in love with death: he dreams
this is the song that hums in the veins of the cold,

if you split the skin of ice
you find these streams of sound.

Then he turns, sighs, remembers the owl
that nests in the stone chimney,

its note the true
question of astonishment,

the question that
broods inside the music.

4
I ask you to meet me outside the house
in that clearing where the birches
circle like ceremonial candles.

You say no, you won't, you
can't be there. At dawn
I go anyway.

Beethoven's waiting,
he's waited all night, his enormous
thicket of hair is wet.

But he smiles. Wide-awake, leaning
against a white-faced tree,
smiles and recites

the single diminished
seventh
of his own death.

The Mothers at Seventy

This one wears her emeralds to bed, that one
spends afternoons in the linen closet
fingering the old quilts, the sheets worn
thin as kleenex.
                    This one
swallows goblets of cream, splashes her hair
with yellow feathers, flings her children's poems
into the sea off Cap d'Antibes.
                                    That one
clamps the shadows down with tacks, munches dust, draws
a tub of acid, whimpering *pain, pain.*

I see them opposite me, two women
waiting on the far shore of a summer lake.
Waiting, watching, they saunter along a grassy path
among heavy hemlocks. One is sprightly, one limps,
one in flowers, one in a gray veil.

I am the star camper, the captain of the swim team.
I show off my strokes, my power, the fancy
flash of my tan. Slowly, proudly
I swim toward them
through the blue egg of my life.

Marriage

—FOR E.

Music remembers: that Mozart
duet in which we met, and hours
of Mahler, Wagner, Strauss—

crimson-plush-upholstered concert halls
around the world
where you conducted me through rondos, intermezzi, arias

of superhuman fervor.
The grass outside Bayreuth! The ragged postwar Germans,
    the lobster
at the interval, all sauced with gilt

and guilt! You the rakish Don, I
the tender ear you nibbled. . . .
It was a major key, you and me!

Now Chicago, and the echoing
shell by the waves: Beethoven's
promises of triumph, Ives's hesitations.

Beyond the winding drive along the shore,
the handsome houses, the aesthetes,
the lake spreads atonal mysteries,

black and blank and pure.
Are you still Giovanni, am I still
Zerlina? Odd halves

and quarters of our voices
hiss on the beach. Music
crawls by us on the water,

recalls us, opens its dark
flanks, calls us to ourselves,
to ghostly chords, archaic harmonies.

Anniversary Waltz

—FOR E.

Talking to you is as embarrassing as talking
to myself: I think everyone will stare, they'll say
Look at that crazy lady, muttering
Love, Love, like a lunatic!

We stoop together in the garden,
stuck in gummy cabbage patches,
nagging, laughing, cursing. When you look up,
I admire your eyebrows, as always.

Satanic, magisterial, Jewish!
I used to dream myself to sleep picturing your eyebrows
raised in my direction!
Yet soon enough we moved into a German ballroom

with bamboo partitions.
You wrote your famous letter to the I.G.
Senators wrote to us.
Our firstborn baby died.

Twenty-one years went by.
More children, more kitchens, better partitions.
Typewriters, studies, weeping in the pantry.
Making love like adolescents on the sly.

Your beard begins to get gray,
but not your eyebrows.
We're stuck in the thick of it, we smile wryly,
we fatten, we grow dumb.

Once in a while
I have to hang on to your hand.
I cannot imagine who else
we might have become.

Rain/Insomnia/North Coast

There are nights when the rain on the roof
writes a cold braille of promises
as if no one were listening, no one
ever meant to listen.

The rain speaks in a small intermittent
code of holes
with absolute indifference
like a message from one star to another.

They're quiet up there, and perfectly busy,
shifting spaces, never judging
our weaknesses, our headaches,
our nights of waking.

You and I lie like twin fevers
under the sheets, trying to get well, trying
to figure out those sentences
not meant to speak to us.

We think we've drunk too much, we think
we're imagining things again:
but when we doze, our four walls
sink deeper into somebody else's thoughts

and a tide of voices
closes over the roof;
asleep, we lapse into moisture,
let go of each other, give up our headaches.

It's gray outside, and misty.
The tongues of silence are growing like kelp.
All night they lick our windows, all night
the drowned house

creeps through the fields toward the sea.

After Thanksgiving

Lord, as Rilke says, the year bears down toward winter, past
the purification of the trees, the darkened brook.
Only 4:45, and the sky's sheer black
clasps two clear planets and a skinny moon
as we drive quietly home from the airport,
the last kid gone.

The time of preparation's over, the time of
harvesting the seed, the husk, the kernel, saving
what can be saved—weaves of sun like
rags of old flannel, provident peach stones,
pies, pickles, berry wines to
hold the sweetness for a few more months.

Now the mountains will settle into their old
cold habits, now the white
birch bones will rise
like all those thoughts we've tried to repress:
madness of the solstice, phosphorescent
logic that rules the fifteen-hour night!

Our children, gorged, encouraged, have taken off
in tiny shuddering planes. Plump with stuffing,
we too hurry away, holding hands, holding on.
Soon it'll be January, soon snow will
shuffle down, cold feathers, swathing us in
inches of white silence—

and the ways of the ice
will be narrow, delicate.

On the Train

All day we chugged into history, past
the redwood cabins with sliding doors and parasols,
the tarmac, the heaps of sawdust, along

that muddy creek the trick motorcyclists always leap,
past the fingers of poison oak, the thornbushes,
the scar on the hill where the burn got out of control.

You gave me a diet pepsi, the children ate cookies,
we told jokes while the train creaked and screeched
between grassy banks as if wild hands

were strangling the engine: over and over
the wheels fell on the tracks like drops of lead
or fistfuls of wet metal.

But as we went the trees became enormous,
the creek cleared, the bushes fattened
and shone with scarlet berries.

And you too were changed, your face
flushed, your beard bloomed and flowed
and darkened like a black geranium.

You were seven feet tall! You smelled of the sea!
And I heard myself say, O my handsome sailor,
come live with me in the splintery shack by the river,

the one that peers like a lover
into the face of the stream,
the one whose flanks are caressed by ferns.

When we came to the old station in the forest
our great-grandfathers were waiting on the platform
dressed in black and looking anxious.

They gave us their blessing,
                              they said it was time
we all began again.

Ponce de León

—FOR E.

In Hallandale and Hollywood
the seventy-year-old Jewish ladies
and their shrunken sneakered husbands

are hurrying out for the Early Bird Specials:
bent, redhaired Emma R., two
sandwiches at a time,

hops to at the Little Rascal,
Yan ladles wontons, Rico flings veal.
The skinny old men eat voraciously,

they eat as though sandwiches and wontons
would keep them alive forever, alive and on the beach,
where I want you to be, you, fifty-three-years-old

now, with your rosy lips and graying beard.
Well, why, when I think of you, do I
think of islands in swamps, Ponce de León places

where your eyes would always glitter?
Let's go back to the early world of the sword grass,
away from the Rascals,

back to the heaving world where the rare blue heron
meditates above water hyacinth
and the marsh hen skids in

for a splashy landing:
it gets dark there at six,
after a flush of rose like yours,

and we'll sleep on a bank like two
bad alligators, two stones.
The fishermen will steer toward us, flashlights

glinting, then turn back:
Don't disturb the Seminoles.
These are the old people,

the ones who were here when
the buzzards first took flight
and the world began.

It's 2085, you're walking on a dirt road
in Sicily, you're my blood-
kin, a seventeen-year-old girl

with black curls and a faint smudge of
shadow on your upper lip.
                              Have you

come from New York to find lost ancestors,
or have you always been here?
Dry hills, stacks of heat,

tower around you; nearby, there are goats, donkeys, chickens,
a smell of dung simmering,
and smoke, grain, *rosmarino;*

in the sky, a track of supersonic light—
but you don't look up, you're reading, thinking,
trying to imagine the past,

and my sentences won't help you, though they
brood in you like chromosomes:
                              I can't

tell you who I was, in my queer costume,
with my modern ideas.
                              My words

stand in the fields beside you—
stones, dead trees—the way
the land you walk through

stood behind me, an unknown monument.
And now the road unfolds and shines ahead
like the history neither of us understands.

It turns you
toward the sea, toward
the inarticulate Aegean.